# Dedication

*This book is dedicated to all the young athletes around the country. You are the future of sports in this country and others, and I want to help make sure that you have an outstanding experience in your respective sports. I want to make sure that you are given the education and skills necessary to make it a long-term commitment if that is your choice. This book is also dedicated to the parents who recognize their child's passion for a sport, and want to help them unleash their potential. Lastly, this is for the hard working coaches, who have so much compassion for their athletes, and who want to see them succeed not only in competition but in life. This book is for all of you, and I hope it serves as a tool for success.*

# CHAPTERS

# 1

# INTRODUCTION

---

Youth athletics is an area that is, in my opinion, severely underserved. Far too many club and high school teams around the country do not even have an athletic trainer or EMT staff present at sporting events. Likewise, many public middle and high schools, especially those in urban areas, do not have an athletic trainer assigned to them. Coaches who are new to coaching, or who are not yet credentialed with a coaching certification (National Coaches Association, National Strength and Conditioning Association, etc), may not be adequately trained to appropriately tailor training for their sport. In addition, most parents are not trained or well versed in training format or injury prevention. Where does this leave the kids? Youth athletes are the most susceptible to injury, poor training, and poor nutrition, and their performance is limited because of this.

The purpose of this book is to educate athletes, parents, and coaches, on the components that factor into the overall performance of the youth athlete. It offers a holistic approach that goes far beyond just physical training, because improving performance and success is not all about lifting heavy weights and running to exhaustion. Ultimately, the goals of youth athletics are to have fun, learn discipline and teamwork, assess talent, and ensure that talent is complemented with safe and appropriate training to allow for a long career in the sport if desired. At the end of this book, the reader will be able to:

- Understand the psychological components associated with sports training, and identify techniques to enhance the mindset of the youth athlete

- Identify common injuries for young athletes, the mechanisms of injury, and the implications on time away from sport, rehab, and return to play

- Learn the non-training ways to help prevent injury in athletes

- Understand what is required in sports nutrition, how nutrition varies depending on the goal and sport, and understand some of the common eating disorders that may arise

- Identify the 8 major components to improving performance through training, implement several exercises and activities in each of these components, and understand the purpose and differences between them

- Learn how to implement periodization in order to maximize peak performance, and learn how to avoid overtraining and deconditioning

# 2

# IT'S ALL MENTAL

This may be the most important chapter in the book. Everyone has heard the saying, "sports are 80% mental, and 20% physical". Well there is a great deal of truth in that statement. Optimal physical training begins with a strong foundation of habits formed through developing a positive mindset, discipline, and goal setting.

# Eliminating Negativity, Focusing on the Positive

An athlete can improve his or her performance by focusing on things that elicit positivity. This may mean changing the friends with whom he or she associates. Adolescence is a time where people can be easily influenced by their friends, and a need for social acceptance is at its peak. There are many stories of athletes with tremendous talent who never "made it big" because they fell into the wrong crowd. Underage drinking, illegal drug abuse, and skipping school are just a few of the negative factors. Bullying has also become a major issue in recent years, and it plays a significant part in the psychological health of an adolescent.

Negativity can also come from family members and coaches. "Why are you growing your hair so long?" "Do you have to wear those type of clothes?" "You ran that race totally wrong and that's why you lost. Do you just like losing?" "Why did you let that kid push right past you and sack your quarterback? You are so weak!" Sometimes parents and coaches can be too critical of their athletes, even though their intentions are not malicious. That being said, these kinds of comments can create a cycle of negative thoughts in the athlete's mind, making it even harder for them to visualize success.

Ensuring that these athletes are surrounded by positive influences can prevent the cycles of negativity that lead to poor performance. Constructive criticism, given in a way to help improve performance instead of highlighting mistakes, promotes positive feedback. Keeping an eye on the friends and acquaintances surrounding the athlete to ensure they are staying safe and doing the right things, is also critical.

# Controlling the Subconscious Mind

This may sound a little "hocus pocus", but we are all capable of creating success, whether it be in business, relationships, athletics, or anything else, by controlling what we feed our subconscious mind. The subconscious mind is that part of us that stores impulses and thoughts that we feed it on a daily basis. It gathers these thoughts and, over time, habits and attitudes are formed. The subconscious mind will respond to negative thoughts just as easily as positive thoughts. If an athlete is told by his father over and over again that he will never be good enough to be a starter, or if his friends tell him he isn't fast enough, these negative thoughts will be stored in his subconscious mind. As the negativity continues, his subconscious mind will cause him to start believing that he is inadequate, and this will show in his performance.

Likewise, if he is surrounded by supportive parents with encouraging words, friends who stay late after practice to help him with drills, and coaches that ensure he has adequate practice, his subconscious mind will absorb all of this positivity. He, too will have to stimulate his subconscious mind by giving himself "pep talks". This creates a subconscious mind full of positivity, which promotes success.

The thing to remember is that the subconscious mind will take in negative impulses just as readily as it will the positive ones. The impulses that fill up the most space in the subconscious mind will win overall and will be manifested in the athlete's overall attitude toward his or her self. Athletes who have a positive outlook on their training and themselves will have much greater success in their athletic endeavors.

# Turning Rituals Into Habits

Mentally preparing for a big competition doesn't just start the night before. It is developed over time by creating rituals that form into habits. The characteristic that sets elite and professional athletes high above the average competitor, is discipline. They have created a series of rituals throughout their day to help them prepare. These rituals should be positive, and should be followed every day in order to form the habit of good practice. A good morning ritual may be to wake up at the first sound of the alarm, get dressed and go for a run, come back and listen to positive music while getting ready, eat breakfast, and head off to school. If this is repeated every day, it will become habit. That means that even if the athlete decides to hang out with friends the night before, she will still wake up the next day and perform the same ritual. Positive rituals promote success, and they eliminate inconsistency, poor eating, and negative thought.

Parents can help their children by assisting them with creating a schedule to complete all of their tasks. This may include setting time for practicing their sport, doing homework, finishing household chores, and setting aside time to meet with friends. A well balanced schedule that includes adequate times for work and play will optimize positivity and success in performance.

Coaches can also aid in creating habits by holding athletes responsible and accountable for their attendance at practice. Taking attendance at the beginning of every practice is a great tool for teaching accountability, as well as time management. Consequences for tardiness should be implemented in a way that reinforces positive behavior. For example, have the athlete write her goals for the season on paper and bring it to the next practice. Hopefully, this will cause her to think about the necessary actions she will need to take in order to achieve those goals, including coming to practice on time! This will also help the coach in tailoring workouts to better prepare the athlete to meet these goals.

# Visualization

In basketball, shooters talk about how they can see the shot going in before the ball leaves their hands. In football, receivers visualize catching the ball for the game winning touchdown. World class runners "see" themselves over and over pacing the perfect race and sprinting to the finish. Visualization is another way of promoting positive thoughts for the subconscious mind. If an athlete cannot imagine himself crossing the finish line first, the likelihood of it happening in real life is decreased. Some athletes have been known to will themselves to victory just by visualizing it. UFC (Ultimate Fighting Championships) Champion, Conor McGregor, was interviewed prior to his match that won him the title belt against Jose Aldo in late 2015. In that interview, he said that he had visualized himself catching Aldo off guard in a short knockout style fight. His visualizations were right on, as he knocked out Aldo only seconds into the fight to win the title! Visualization is one of the most powerful tools in the mental preparation needed for success.

# Set Goals

As mentioned earlier, setting goals is a way to hold the athlete accountable. It also makes achieving something visualized even more realistic once it is written down on paper. Having the athlete think of what he or she wants to accomplish this season will give not only the athlete, but the parents and coaches an idea of the work that needs to be done. Keep in mind, these goals need to be measurable, specific, and should have a time frame for completion.

Once these goals are written, have the athlete put them in a place where they can be read daily. A good, private place may be right above the athlete's bed, or in a journal they can read every night. The more the goals are read, the more real they become, and the subconscious mind begins to believe them as true. Once that happens, success is soon to follow!

Many successful business men and women say that they write their goals down every day. The goals may change, or stay the same. However, they almost never scale down the goals. If an athlete sets a goal of hitting 15 home runs in a season, but has never hit more than 2 in any season prior, that is ok. Just know that in order to achieve the goal, far more work may be needed to achieve it than was done in previous seasons. If the athlete is willing to put forth the effort needed to make it happen, then it will likely be accomplished. The moral of the story is, don't change the goal, change the actions that will lead to achieving the goal!

# Make it Fun

Whether they are ten or twenty, young athletes want to have fun! Being talented enough to compete in a sport is a privilege and a reward. It should not feel like work. It is a known fact that people work harder, and are more self-driven, when they are passionate about something, and when it is fun. Allowing the athlete to choose in which sport he or she wants to participate is a start. Giving rewards for good performance (a personal best time, game winning goal, etc) and decreasing the negative comments will also maintain the "fun" factor. There is a difference between a child who does not wish to play a certain sport, and a child who is interested in the sport but not disciplined to do the work needed to improve performance. Creating rituals and habits for the latter is the best way to address the undisciplined child. For the child who is just not interested in the sport, find another sport or activity! Forcing kids to participate in sports or activities in which they are not interested can lead to a whole other set of problems.

Physical readiness to compete is only a small part of the equation. Aside from talents received from birth and physical training, success in sports is the direct result of creating a positive mindset, implementing rituals that create habits, visualization, and having fun. Setting goals and writing them down serves as the bridge between thinking positively and making it a reality. All of these actions create belief, and that is the underlying key to success. Belief is what inspires people to do one more rep of squats, stay 10 more minutes after practice to work on heading the ball, and take one more practice start out of the blocks. With a positive mindset and strong belief, the athlete is ready for any competition and programmed for victory!

# 3
# COMMON SPORTS INJURIES IN ADOLESCENTS

Children and adolescents deal with some of the same types of injuries as adults, but some injuries are more common and specific to the 10-20 year old population. This chapter describes several of these injuries, and gives the reader information on post-injury treatment options. It also describes the impact on the athlete returning to competition.

# Osgood-Schlatter Disorder

This is injury affects the knees. The onset usually occurs during a period of rapid growth, somewhere around the start of puberty. The growth plates just below the kneecap (on the tibial tubercle) become inflamed as the child's body is not able to keep up with the rate of growth. Pain may begin only after practicing or competition. As inflammation progresses, the athlete may start to report pain that occurs both during and after activity. A proper exam by a physician is recommended to rule out any other pathologies. The physician may recommend physical therapy for 3 to 4 weeks to control symptoms and for education on safe strengthening of the knee. Acute management of Osgood-Schlatter includes icing several times per day, as well as decreased activity for at least 3 to 4 weeks (or until symptoms subside). During this time, participation in sport should be minimized, with no intense practices or competitions while healing. The athlete may be ready to return to sport when pain is no longer elicited during and after activity, and when no signs of compensatory movements with activity are observed (limping, avoiding pushing off of the affected leg, etc).

# Ankle Sprain

This is one of the most common injuries for children and adults. The term "sprain" implies that an overstretching occurs to one or more ligaments of the ankle, either from a "rolling in" or "rolling out" motion. The more common type of ankle sprain is the "rolling in", or inversion sprain. Ice should be applied within the first 5 minutes of injury, and the athlete should be assisted to a seat to rest, preferably with the leg elevated higher than the level of the heart. Swelling frequently occurs with an ankle sprain, however the degree varies. It is also important to keep in mind that the degree of swelling does not indicate the severity of the sprain. The athlete should be taken for x-rays to make sure there is no fracture of the ankle, and for crutches if necessary. Physical therapy may also be recommended for balance and stability training for the ankle. The length of time out of competition depends on the severity of the sprain, and can range from 2 weeks to several months. Grade III ankle sprains are the most severe and may need surgical intervention to repair. If surgery is recommended, the rehab process will be much longer.

# Shoulder Dislocation

Shoulder dislocations are more common in adolescents than adults. Adults tend to have shoulder pain and injury from a "stiffening" of the shoulder due to arthritis and other conditions caused by worsening posture. Dislocations are usually caused by one of two things...1. The athlete is "born loose" (hypermobile) and predisposed to injury, or 2. The athlete has a direct contact injury to the shoulder. If the athlete is "born loose", dislocation can occur just from raising the arm overhead, without any weight in hand. If there is a direct contact injury, it usually occurs with the arm out to the side at shoulder level, and outwardly rotated (as in a throwing motion). With a contact injury, there is a risk for fracture, so immediate medical care is recommended for x-rays and exam by a physician. In either case, physical therapy is recommended to regain range of motion, strengthen, and stabilize the muscles surrounding the shoulder complex. The average length of rehab is 2-3 months. Rehab after surgical intervention can be 6-9 months depending on the severity of injury.

# Elbow Fracture

Elbow fractures in adolescents usually occur from falling with an outstretched arm, as if to break the fall. The most common type of fracture is closed, which means the bone has not broken the skin. In most cases, these fractures do not require surgery to heal, and the athlete is usually casted for 6-8 weeks. Following removal of the cast, the athlete will undergo 2-3 months of therapy before easing back into sport. Another common type of fracture is an open fracture, in which the bone breaks through the skin. The risk of infection is higher in these fractures, and surgery is required. Therefore, the length of time for healing and rehab is longer, usually a minimum of 3-6 months.

# Medial Collateral Ligament Tear of the Elbow

This injury is common to athletes in throwing sports, primarily baseball pitchers. The mechanics of an overhead thrower are vital, and any abnormal mechanics or overuse through excessive throwing can put the athlete at risk for this type of injury. If the ligament tear is severe, surgery may be recommended. The most common type of surgery for an MCL (medial collateral ligament) tear in the elbow is the "Tommy John" surgery. Healing time following surgery is 6-8 weeks, followed by a minimum of 3-6 months of therapy before returning to play. Upon return to play, throwing reps should be carefully monitored so as not to cause re-injury.

# Quadriceps and Hamstrings Strains

These are lower extremity injuries that typically occur in sports such as track and field (mostly sprinting), where the athlete is accelerating to top speed very quickly. The more common of the two injuries is a strain of the hamstrings, usually because the hamstrings are a smaller muscle group and are typically not trained as much as the quadriceps group. Ice should be applied within the first several minutes of a strain and throughout the acute phase of the injury (within the first 24 to 48 hours). Following the acute phase, heat may be used along with compression to keep the leg "warm" and maintain flexibility. A contrast of alternating cold and heat is also used, each lasting about 3-5 minutes, to promote healthy blood flow and speed the healing process. Light stretching will also help with flexibility. A progression of strengthening and dynamic stretching, as well as manual therapy can be initiated by an athletic trainer or physical therapist. Typically, the length of rehab is about 4 to 6 weeks.

Less commonly, an athlete can have a strain of one or more of the four quadriceps tendons. The largest of the four is the rectus femoris, and severe injury to this muscle can also result in a fracture to the bony attachment on the pelvis. The injury is caused by excessive force to the quads with sprinting or any activity that works the hip flexors. Recovery time depends on the extent of the strain, but can be as little as 3 to 4 weeks. If a fracture of the pelvis is involved, the athlete may be non-weightbearing for 4-6 weeks, followed by 2-3 months of therapy to strengthen and stabilize the hip and/or knee. Core strengthening is also essential with this injury due to the proximity of the quads and hamstrings to the lower core muscles.

# Patellofemoral Pain

Patellofemoral pain (PTF pain) is common in athletes who participate in sports requiring frequent jumping, such as basketball, volleyball, and track and field athletes competing in the jumps (long jump, triple jump, and high jump) and hurdles.  For this reason, it is often referred to as "jumper's knee".  Patellofemoral pain is often a chronic pain felt over the patellar tendon, just below the kneecap.  This occurs from repetitive overuse, most commonly from frequent jumping or running.  This condition does not require surgery, but rehab with physical therapy can be prolonged due to the chronic nature of the condition. Many coaches and parents do not like to hear it, but the best therapy for PTF pain to subside is REST!  Rehab may take 6-8 weeks, followed by a scheduled transition back to full competition.

# ACL Tears

The anterior cruciate ligament is the most common ligament tear in the knee. It can occur from a direct trauma to the knee, but it often occurs when the athlete has the foot planted while trying to change directions. The medial collateral ligament may also be sprained in the injury, but a sprain to the MCL most times does not require surgery. However, ACL tears commonly require surgery, especially if the athlete intends to continue competing. Rehab and return to play is, at a minimum, 9 months. Many athletes say that they feel "back to normal" at about the 3 to 4 month mark in their rehab. However, this feeling of "strength" occurs because of the healing process of the ACL. There is initial strength in the new ACL in the first several days following surgery, followed by a period of weakness that may last several months. Most athletes start to regain a significant amount of muscular strength by the 3-4 month mark, even though the ACL itself is still in a period of weakness and healing. Returning to high intensity activity at this time can put the athlete at great risk for re-injury.

Female athletes are at a significantly higher risk for ACL tear due to the nature of their anatomy. The female knee is shaped with more of a valgus posture (a more "knee-kneed" position), and the space between the two bones that make up the knee joint (the femur and tibia) is narrower than in males. These two differences put the ACL in a position where it absorbs more stress and forces from regular knee motions, and these forces are intensified with running, jumping, and cutting movements.

There are several different grafts that can be used to reconstruct the ACL, including a cadaver ACL, patellar tendon, hamstring tendon, and the gastrocnemius tendon. The two most common grafts are the cadaver ACL and patellar tendon. There are differences in rehab strategies early in the rehab process, but overall the length of time to return to play is about the same (9 to 12 months). Returning to controlled strength and conditioning and sport-specific drills can begin at about the 6 month mark depending on how well the athlete is progressing. Pain at the 6-month period is an indication not to return to play.

# Stress Fractures

Most commonly occurring in the bones of the feet and shins (tibias), stress fractures are small fractures of the bone that occur from overuse. Cross country runners are especially at risk for developing stress fractures due to the long distance running that occurs frequently. Overuse injuries such as this can occur from two common problems. First, stress fractures can occur from overtraining without adequate periods of decreased intensity and rest in training. Correct programming and periodization of a competition season should allow for periods of at least 3-4 weeks where training is significantly decreased to allow time for healing. The second common reason for stress fracture development is when an athlete returns to intense activity after being deconditioned. In this case, the athlete did not have sufficient training during the "off-season" or is coming back from injury and simply doing too much too soon. Running 3 miles at one time after not running at all for 3 months is a recipe for disaster!

Similarly to PTF pain syndrome, the length of time for recovery from stress fractures is longer due to the chronic nature of the injury. Surgery is typically not required, but the athlete may be placed in a walking boot for 4-6 weeks in order to relieve pressure on the foot with walking, and walking should be limited. Physical therapy rehab can then take an additional 6 to 8 weeks for strengthening and stabilization.

# Concussion

This is a topic that has seen a lot of attention in recent years, particularly in the NFL and college football. Concussion management is especially important in youth athletics, where athletes may not have the resources and sports medicine team available.

Concussions are caused by traumatic head injury, either from direct contact with another athlete, or from hitting the head on a hard surface. There are levels of severity of concussion, varying from minimal dizziness or lightheadedness, to temporary unconsciousness. All sports teams should be equipped with a concussion check off sheet that can be obtained from the team trainer or local EMT unit. Some of the more serious signs of concussion that require immediate medical attention include memory loss, blurred vision, slurred speech, bleeding from the ears or nose, and severe headache lasting greater than 72 hours. It is easy to overlook less severe symptoms of concussion, such as tenderness at the site of impact, temporary confusion, and lightheadedness. However, coaches and parents need to be advocates for the athletes and allow them time to rest. A good rule of thumb to follow is, "when in doubt, sit them out." Time out from sport for concussion can be as little as one week, to more than a month. The athlete should be screened by a trained concussion management professional, such as an MD, PT, or athletic trainer. Concussions should be taken very seriously, as symptoms can manifest years after the athlete is done competing. Long-term effects of memory loss, decreased concentration, and Parkinson's-like symptoms can be devastating.

# 4

# INJURY PREVENTION

Having the proper training program is essential in optimizing performance with any sport. However, taking the right steps to prevent injuries is equally as important. Injury prevention is a collaborative effort and must involve the athlete, parents, and coaches.

# Warm-up

Before practicing or before a competition, an adequate set of stretches and exercises is required to warm-up the athlete's muscle tissues and prepare him or her for intense physical activity. Traditional warm-ups have included an active exercise, such as running or biking, followed by static stretching. However, recent research and training programs have moved toward an all-active warm-up, consisting of an active exercise (jogging, biking, stair stepper, treadmill walking) followed by active or dynamic stretching.

Static stretching, such as the traditional seated hamstring stretch, consists of the athlete obtaining the stretch position for the intended muscle group, and then holding that position for about 30 seconds without moving. Active, or dynamic stretching, involves stretching the intended muscles group with a movement exercise that safely moves the muscles through a range from a stretched position to a shortened, or contracted, position. For example, walking high leg kicks is a dynamic stretch for the hamstrings.

Both static and dynamic stretches are good for a warm-up, but the reason for choosing one over the other may depend on the flexibility of the athlete. Athletes who are naturally flexible tend to do well with static and dynamic stretching, and have an easier time warming-up their muscle tissues. Athletes who naturally have decreased flexibility or are "stiff", may respond better to an active exercise followed by dynamic stretching versus static stretching. Warming-up with static stretching only is not recommended for athletes with limited flexibility. This is because these athletes are placing more strain on their muscles to get into stretch positions, and static stretching can put them at risk for injury (tear or muscle strain). It's similar to trying to stretch out a very thick rubber band with a lot of resistance versus a thin rubber band that can easily be expanded. If that thick rubber band is stretched too far too fast, it can break. The same thing can happen if an inflexible athlete is trying to perform static stretching on cold, stiff muscles. Active exercise and dynamic stretching provide a higher level of blood flow to the muscles and provide a safer way to warm-up the body in preparation for the high demand placed upon it with intense training.

Another important consideration for choosing a proper warm-up deals with the type of activity that is going to be performed. If the workout is only aerobic (cardio) or low to moderate resistance training, a short active warm-up with static or dynamic stretching is usually adequate. However, if the athlete is going to be performing any exercises that require explosive movements (power, agility, plyometric, etc), a dynamic warm-up is preferred. These activities require the muscles to move through an entire movement (such as a squat jump) either with high velocity, heavy weight, or both. During the movement, the muscles will have to change from a shortened or contracted position, to a stretched position, in a short amount of time. Using dynamic stretching and warm-up exercises better prepares the muscles and joints for the extreme stretch-contract movements. Static stretching does not provide enough preparation since the muscles are held in one position (the stretched position) the entire duration of the stretch.

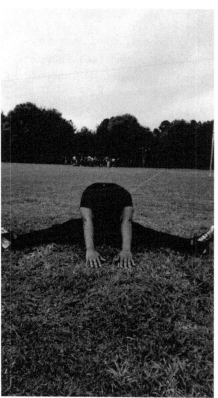

Seated hamstring stretch

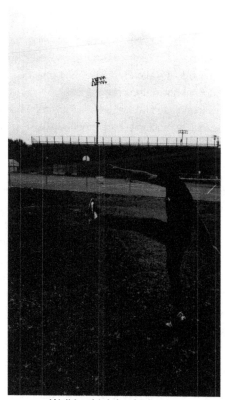

Walking high leg kicks

# Cool Down

Light exercise and stretching following intense training, especially after anaerobic training, can help to prevent cramping and muscle soreness. Unlike the warm-up, the athlete's muscles are already "loose" and may be hypertrophied due to training. Hypertrophy occurs due to the breaking of blood capillaries in the muscle fibers, a natural occurrence with intense physical activity. It is as if the muscles are inflamed on a low grade scale. Static stretching is recommended post-activity to decrease heart rate, decrease risk of cramping, and "cool down" the muscle tissues. Some athletes may also benefit from icing, especially if they are recovering from injury or tend to overheat with exercise.

Warm-ups and cool-downs should be group or team activities, for several different reasons. First, it builds camaraderie and teamwork, which is important in "team sports" such as football, soccer, and lacrosse. Sports such as track and field are considered "individual" sports, so building this team atmosphere helps not only during championship season when each individual effort counts towards the total team score, but it also helps to build the teamwork skills needed in all facets of life. Secondly, it builds congruency and standardizes the stretching program. If someone is late to practice, he or she can still go through the warm-up process, hopefully with a partner, because the exercises and routine is known by everyone on the team. Lastly, doing the warm-up and cool-down in a group/ team manner allows the coaches to monitor their athletes to ensure that exercises are not only being done, but that they are being done right. This will eliminate the risk of injury from a lack of stretching or from improper stretching.

# Overtraining

Far too often, young athletes develop injuries from overtraining by coaches and parents. Every sport has a training cycle, and the cycle should include a period about midway through the season where practice sessions are tapered down. Constant high-intensity training can quickly lead to overtraining, and can have a deteriorating effect on performance. If an athlete shows a decline in performance for several consecutive competitions, chances are he or she is suffering from overtraining.

Not only can overtraining cause a decline in performance, it can also put the athlete at risk for injury. Common overtraining injuries in long distance runners include IT Band friction syndrome, stress fracture, and patellofemoral pain. In football, overtraining injuries can include hamstring strain, turf toe, and MCL/ACL sprain.

No matter the sport, each training program should have a workout schedule that cycles between high-intensity days and low to medium intensity days. This includes not only sport specific training, but any resistance and weight lifting program that may complement individual sport training. Athletes should not train more than 6 days per week, with a 7th day free of any training to allow the body time to recover. Some strength and conditioning coaches recommend a very light form of exercise, usually jogging, on the 7th day, to keep the "blood flowing". However, there will be no negative effect on performance with not doing any exercise. Athletes who are involved in more than one sport or who play on more than one team, are better served using that seventh day as a complete rest day.

# Heat Exhaustion/Heat Stroke

As mentioned previously, some athletes may overheat with intense physical activity. This is especially true for athletes who live in warmer climates, such as Florida, Texas, and California. Outdoor practices may last 2 to 3 hours, and sporting events such as track meets can last all day. In humid climates, the effects of the heat is more evident and draining on the body. However, in dryer climates the heat can be more harmful, even deadly, because it is not as easily noticed. It is important to make sure athletes are resting in a shaded area in between competitions to prevent prolonged exposure to the sun.

Signs of heat exhaustion include lack of perspiration, disorientation, light headedness, and confusion. If heat exhaustion is suspected, the athlete should be taken to a shaded area, or indoors to an air conditioned space. Using ice (or cold water if no ice is available) can be placed all over the body to help cool the athlete's body temperature, starting with the carotid and radial pulses first (neck and wrist). Heat stroke is more serious than heat exhaustion and can cause complete disorientation to person, place, and time. The athlete can even become unconscious. Immediate medical attention is required for suspected heat stroke.

# Hydration

Proper hydration is vital for optimizing performance. The vast majority of athletes are highly under-hydrated. Hydration comes not only from water intake, but all fluids consumed throughout the day. Water is, of course, the most essential fluid for replenishing the body's fluid levels lost through sweating. Sports drinks, such as Gatorade and Powerade, are also vital to replace some of the key electrolytes lost through sweating and physical activity. These electrolytes include sodium chloride, potassium, magnesium, and calcium. Sodium chloride is the major electrolyte lost during sweating.

In order to formally measure sweat loss, the athlete's weight should be measured before activity, and then again after activity. If the athlete has greater than 2% of their body weight lost after activity, this indicates dehydration. More than a 2-3% weight loss through loss of fluids can raise the body's core temperature, creating overheating and fatigue throughout the body. The athlete will most likely complain of being thirsty and may have a lack of perspiration. Electrolyte loss can lead to cramping and decreased strength, accuracy, and endurance when training.

The amount of hydration needed to maintain optimal levels in the body varies from athlete to athlete, based on weight and each athlete's tendency to sweat more or less. Water consumption before and during exercise can prevent dehydration. At least six to eight 16oz glasses of water per day is required to maintain adequate hydration in most teenage athletes. This amount may decrease in younger and smaller athletes such as gymnasts, and increase in older and larger athletes such as linemen in football.

Excess loss of electrolytes through sweat can also lead to nausea, vomiting, and headaches. Sports drinks containing electrolytes are most efficient when consumed during intense training lasting more than 1 to 2 hours, and after intense physical activity. Water is best consumed before and during activity. When a competition is approaching, the athlete should hydrate the night before and several hours before the competition with water.  Alternating between water and sports drinks during the day of competition is optimal.

# Sleep

Sleep is one of the most overlooked areas for preventing injury. Sleep allows the body time to recover from a hard physical practice, mentally draining day of tests and homework, and emotional stress from a feud with friends. With adequate sleep, the human body is able to repair itself naturally without the use of pain medicines, topical ointments, or supplements. It is recommended that athletes between the ages of 10 and 20 obtain at least 8 to 10 hours of sleep per night. A common misconception is that sleep can be "made up" days later for time missed earlier in the week. This is not true. The body responds to the length of sleep it obtains at that moment, and this has no effect on any sleep, or lack of sleep, obtained in the future. Therefore, sleeping only 6 hours one night and then 12 the next night does not "average" to 9 hours of sleep per night!

If an athlete is getting less than the recommended sleep, he or she will most likely show signs of increased muscle soreness that can last days after intense practices. Decreased sleep can also lead to overeating, as the athlete is staying up longer than required and will seek food to keep her energy levels high.

Having adequate sleep gives the body time to reach the entire Rapid Eye Movement (REM) cycle, allowing for healing and recovery to take place. If an athlete is sleeping too few hours per night to achieve this REM cycle, he or she may complain of waking up tired, and will fatigue quickly throughout the day. This can affect not only performance in sporting activities, but also in the classroom. Inadequate sleep causes lack of concentration and decreased alertness. When trying to perform an intense physical activity, he or she may also experience muscle cramping and fatigue.

# 5

# SPORTS NUTRITION

Nutrition for athletes differs from the nutrition of more sedentary individuals. While the FDA (Food and Drug Administration) bases their nutritional facts on a diet consisting of 2000 calories per day, the typical athlete is most likely consuming well over 2000 calories to meet the demands of his or her training. Likewise, adolescents need to consume more than the prescribed caloric intake per day to meet the demands of growth and development, in addition to any requirements for a specific sport. The exact caloric intake depends on the weight and age of the athlete, the sport in which he or she is competing, and the goal or desired output (weight gain, weight loss, strength gains, muscle hypertrophy, etc). All meal plans will include varying proportions of protein, carbohydrates, and fats. Like the total calorie consumption, the proportions of proteins, carbohydrates, and fats will also depend on the size of the athlete and the desired outcome. The suggested requirements below are general estimates. In order to obtain a specific breakdown and meal plan for an athlete, one should seek the assistance of a registered dietician.

# Protein

Protein is the key to improving performance, and an optimal amount of protein in the daily meal plan can not only help promote weight gain and muscle hypertrophy, but also weight loss. Proteins are made up of amino acids, which are the building blocks and key to maintaining cell structure and function. They help to build and repair the cells of the body, and essential amino acids help to repair the cells of skeletal muscles. Having the correct proportion of protein at each meal gives the athlete an optimal environment in the cells to properly recover from intense training sessions. Consuming about 10-12 grams of protein per meal is ideal, but athletes looking to gain more muscle mass may need to consume about 20 grams per meal. This equates to roughly 15-20% of the daily nutritional intake per day.

The source of the protein consumed will also have an effect on overall performance. Proteins that are low in fat and sodium are better than those with higher levels. For example, having turkey sausage or egg whites at breakfast is better than having pork bacon. Eating chicken breast for lunch is better than eating fried chicken. Eating tilapia or salmon is better than eating catfish or shrimp. Athletes who are vegan or non-meat eaters may need to add a little extra fat to their diet because they are not getting the fats that are naturally contained in meats. Some good sources of vegetarian proteins include soy, tofu, lentil beans, black beans, and chick peas. Snacks that are good sources of protein include raw almonds, string cheese, and Greek yogurt.

# Carbohydrates

Carbohydrates are the primary energy source in the diet. They are what help get a student through a long day of classes, and then become the star athlete who is then called upon to endure a grueling practice. Carbohydrates are broken down into 3 general categories— monosaccharides (simple sugars), disaccharides, and polysaccharides. These types of carbs differ in terms of how quickly they are absorbed in the body to be used as energy. Carbohydrates that are absorbed in the body more slowly are preferred because they reduce the need for the body to release more blood glucose. Rising blood glucose levels can lead to diabetes if they remain high chronically. Simple sugars, or monosaccharides, commonly found in soft drinks and candy, are most likely to cause spikes in blood glucose.

As stated above, when choosing the best carbohydrates to fuel the body, slow absorbing, more complex carbs are preferred. The way in which certain foods are processed can also affect how they are absorbed in the body. Examples include—eating brown rice vs white rice, whole wheat bread vs white bread, sweet potato vs white potato, oatmeal vs cereal. The average carbohydrate consumption for young athletes is between 45-55% of the total diet per day, which is typically about 20-25 grams per meal. Keep in mind that these should be "good" carbs, not added sugars like those found in soft drinks and juices.

# Fats

The third component in every meal is fat. The three primary types of fat either found in the body or consumed, are triglycerides, saturated fats, and unsaturated fats. All of them are composed of different types of fatty acids, which are used in the body to maintain cellular health and function. Of the 3, triglycerides are the "best" type of fat to consume, followed by unsaturated fats. On average, an athlete's meal plan should include about 10-15% fat per day, which is about 6-10 grams per meal. If an athlete is eating more than this amount of fat in his or her diet, the body will not be able to break down all of it and the fat will be stored in the body as adipose tissue.

Obviously, some sources of fat are better than others because they can be broken down and react in the body better. Fish that are high in omega-3 and omega-6 fatty acids are optimal, and can be found in salmon, soy, and corn. Tuna, halibut, and trout also contain these omega-3 fatty acids. One of my favorites, tilapia, is actually fairly low in fat and is an excellent source of protein. Chicken breast and ground turkey meat are also preferred sources of fat from meat versus beef or pork. Olives, nuts, and seeds (sunflower, safflower) are good vegetarian sources of fat.

# Vegetables

Vegetables are another essential element in the diet. Dark green vegetables are the most essential because they contain healthy vitamins and iron, both of which are vital to everyday functions in the body. The athlete should be consuming twice as many vegetables at meal time as he or she is protein and carbs. Examples of dark green veggies include kale, spinach, and field greens. Other green vegetables that provide optimal nutritional value include broccoli, zucchini, and asparagus. Despite popularity, iceberg and romaine lettuce have very little nutritional value. Preparation of these vegetables is also important. Foods that are packaged in cans or foods that are cooked by boiling have much less nutritional value than those that are eaten raw or steamed. Another important fact is that most vegetables are only 30-50 calories per serving, so an athlete can eat more of these to get that "full" feeling instead of eating more protein, carbs or fat.

# Pre and Post Workout/Competition Meals

There has been an ongoing debate as to which is better before workouts. Some professionals say that a meal or snack that is mostly protein is better, and some say a meal or snack that is mostly carbs is better. In my opinion, I believe it has to do with the type of exercise or sport being performed, and the duration. If the duration of physical activity is less than 45 minutes, the sugar from a piece of fruit such as an apple may be sufficient when eaten 30 minutes prior to activity. If the athlete is going to perform the activity for greater than 45 minutes, a meal consisting of both protein and carbs may be more appropriate to ensure that the athlete has enough reserved energy to prevent cramping, fatigue, and prolonged soreness following activity. Immediately following workouts, the athlete should consume at least 12 grams of protein via a protein shake, milk, or meal within 20-30min of the workout. This will help with muscle repair and prevent delayed onset muscle soreness (DOMS).

The night before competition, a meal that is heavy in carbohydrate content is preferred. Many collegiate sports teams have spaghetti or some other type of pasta for dinner the night before a competition, along with the other components of a complete meal (protein, fat, veggies).

For the day of the competition, the athlete should eat a breakfast that is carb heavy. Pancakes, waffles, English muffins, or whole wheat bread are great sources of carbs. Fruits such as apples, oranges, pineapples, and bananas are naturally sweetened and can offer an additional source of carbohydrate, as well as other nutritional benefits (fiber, vitamin C, and potassium). A great way to add an adequate serving of protein to the breakfast is to make protein pancakes, waffles, or muffins! When choosing a breakfast meat, those with lower fat content are preferred (turkey sausage or turkey bacon).

For competitions that last less than one hour, the athlete may only need a snack with healthy carbs, such as orange slices or yogurt. For competitions lasting longer than one hour, such as a track meet, football or basketball game, or all day tournament, there should be ample fruits and yogurt as sources of carbs. The athlete should also have at least one meal that has about 10-15g of protein, such as a peanut butter and jelly sandwich, grilled chicken breast or tuna fish sandwich. Adequate water and electrolyte consumption is also key throughout the day of competition to prevent cramping, fatigue and dehydration.

Overall, athletes must be eating 3 to 4 meals per day with healthy snacks in between. By spacing out the caloric intake throughout the day, the body stays fueled all day long, metabolism stays ramped up, and cravings are decreased. Eating fewer than 3 meals per day, especially without any snacks, can leave the athlete hungry and unfocused during classes. He or she will also feel fatigued when it is time to practice, and bunching those calories together can actually cause metabolism to slow down and create unwanted weight gain.

# Eating Disorders

The two primary eating disorders that are prevalent with young athletes are anorexia nervosa and bulimia nervosa. The underlying cause of both is a negative perception of one's self body image. These illnesses can affect both boys and girls, and may be associated with other psychological disorders such as depression or obsessive-compulsive disorder (OCD). The athlete's mood and self-esteem will be greatly affected with these conditions. Detecting signs of anorexia or bulimia is a team approach including coaches, parents, friends, strength and conditioning coaches, athletic trainers, and doctors. Typically, eating disorders are prevalent in older teenagers and young adults, but it is possible for an athlete younger to experience one or both of these conditions.

Anorexia involves a lack of eating due to fear of gaining weight or already being overweight. The athlete may miss meals, significantly restrict his or her portions, take diet pills or laxatives, or fast. Some athletes with anorexia may be secret binge eaters, and some may binge and purge. Likewise, bulimia involves binge eating with excessive amounts of food, often followed by purging. The athlete may go long periods without eating, and then binge, usually in private.

In addition to changes in eating habits, there are other signs that may indicate an athlete has one or both of these disorders. Mood swings, fatigue and inability to complete workouts, chronic or repetitive injuries, discolored teeth (from purging), and significant weight loss are all signs of eating disorder. In girls, there may be an increase in bleeding or a missed menstrual cycle for one or more months. Intervention is needed with all members of the team collaborating to help the athlete without making him or her feel threatened. The best way to help is to have the athlete speak to a psychologist/psychiatrist.

# 6

# AEROBIC AND RESISTANCE TRAINING

Every sport will have its own sports specific activities and training, whether it's working on fielding ground balls in baseball, perfecting an overhead swing in tennis, or practicing hurdling in track and field. However, no matter the sport in which an athlete is going to participate, there will have to be additional training other than these sport specific skills. Scientific evidence shows that an athlete's performance in a given sport can be improved by adding two essential elements to the training program—aerobic and resistance training.

# Aerobic Training

Aerobic training is the foundation of physical fitness. It allows the body to adapt to changes in the cardiovascular, respiratory, muscular, and endocrine systems that occur with athletic activity. It helps to improve circulation of blood to and from the heart, and optimizes the use of oxygen and transport of different chemicals through the blood. Aerobic exercise also affects the body's metabolic rate (MET), which is a measure of the oxygen demand needed to perform all of the normal functions in the body. Consistent aerobic exercise can affect the athlete's MET by allowing him or her to perform at a higher or more intense level while still being able to perform all of the body's functions. This is how endurance is created.

It is important to consider that with aerobic activity, the athlete will have a rise in heart rate and blood pressure. Normal blood pressure is approximately 120/80, measured in milligrams (mg) of Mercury (Hg). These numbers may be lower in younger children and conditioned athletes, somewhere around 95mg Hg/55mg Hg in some cases. An abnormal response to exercise would be a rise in systolic blood pressure (the top number) by more than 20 mg, or a rise in diastolic blood pressure (the bottom number) more than 10 mg. Another abnormal finding would be a drop by more than 10mg for either systolic or diastolic blood pressure with exercise. Signs of abnormal blood pressure may include complaints of lightheadedness, fainting, or paleness/redness. Every school or team should have a portable wrist blood pressure cuff to take measurements if someone is experiencing these symptoms. In any of these occurrences, exercise needs to be discontinued immediately, and the athlete's primary care physician should be notified.

Another consideration with aerobic exercise is increased heart rate. A rise in heart rate should occur during and immediately following exercise. Following exercise, heart rate should begin to decrease within a minute and should return to a normal range within 2-3 minutes. There is a simple equation to estimate a person's maximal heart rate, the level at which all activity needs to be discontinued. This equation is 220-age (in years). For example, the maximal heart rate for a 15-year old football player would be 205 beats per minute (220-15=205). In my opinion, a young athlete's heart rate should never be greater than 180 bpm. A quick way to check heart rate following an activity is to place the index and middle fingers over the wrist (radial pulse) and count the number of pulses that occur within a 60 second period. Again, if there are any abnormal findings (a drop in heart rate or an increase to the athlete's max level), activity needs to be discontinued and physician notified.

Appropriate aerobic training improves the body's responses to changes in blood pressure and heart rate. Over time with training, the athlete will start to see a decrease in both resting heart rate and blood pressure. There are many types of aerobic activity, and the best way to obtain these long term adaptions to training is to try a combination of aerobic exercise. Technically, any activity lasting longer than 60 seconds is considered aerobic in nature. The athlete can do jumping jacks, jump rope, or run stairs. Some longer durations of exercise may include running, biking, swimming, elliptical machine, or walking on an incline on a treadmill. Aerobic exercise should be performed for a total of 20-30min at least 3-4 times per week in order to optimize results.

# Resistance Training

Resistance training involves moving a body part through all or part of its available range of motion against a resistive force, such as weights, cables, resistance bands/tubes, or other apparatus. It is fundamental to ensuring the muscles of the body are able to keep up with demand placed upon them by physical activity. Resistance exercise can be used for one of three purposes-- muscle strengthening, muscle hypertrophy (increasing the size of the muscles) or tone, and power. Strengthening the muscles also improves stability around the joints, thus decreasing the risk for injury. Exercise programs that include a well-balanced plan incorporating both aerobic and resistance training generally produce higher levels of performance and lower incidences of injury.

When doing resistance exercises for strengthening, the number of repetitions for each exercise will average between 10 and 15, and the athlete can do anywhere from 3 to 5 sets. Weight or resistance selection is based on the amount of effort, and should be between 75-85% of the athlete's maximum effort (1 rep max). In order to gain muscle tone or hypertrophy, the number of reps will increase to 15-20, and the resistance or load will decrease to about 50-70% of the 1 rep max. Resistance training for power involves quick, explosive movements through a range of motion. Power lifts also include multiple muscle groups working through that range of motion, so the athlete is getting more of a total body workout. These exercises will be performed at 85-90% of the 1 rep max, and the athlete will perform anywhere from 4 to 6 reps.

While posture and body mechanics are essential in any type of resistance training, they are particularly imperative with power exercises due to the explosiveness of the exercise against a heavy load. The prevalence of injury is higher in these exercises, such as dead lifts, power cleans, squats, and bench press. When beginning a resistance training program, close monitoring of body mechanics and form is necessary, and should be conducted by the coach (if qualified), athletic or strength trainer for the team. Periodic checks during sessions will also help decrease the risk of injury. Athletes should never lift alone, and a spot must be used with any overhead or squatting activities.

Regarding age appropriateness, resistance training can be included with athletes ages 14 and up. However, children who have just begun puberty should not do resistance training with heavy weights because their joints are still growing and too much stress on the joints can cause abnormal fusing of the growth plates. This can lead to chronic injury and impaired growth. Body weight exercises and calisthenics are recommended for athletes in the younger age range, between 10 and 14. Push-ups, pull-ups, body weight squats, lunges, and abdominal exercises are great examples. An alternative to using weights, if resistance is being used, is to use resistance bands or tubing. This will reduce the amount of stress being placed on the joints while giving resistance throughout the range of motion. With older athletes who may already be in high school, discretion should be used as to whether or not the athlete is ready to begin a resistance training program with increasing weights. Another big issue is the depth at which an athlete squats. If the angle of the knee joint is greater than 90 degrees when squatting, the athlete is adding more shearing forces to the knee and placing increased stress on the ACL. Keeping squat depth to that 90 degree angle is ideal for preventing early wear and tear of the knee joint. Before beginning any resistance training, consulting with a primary care physician, physical therapist, athletic trainer, or strength and conditioning specialist is recommended.

# 7

# SPEED AND AGILITY DRILLS

Strengthening and aerobic exercise are the foundation for physical fitness, but there are other factors to address in order to improve performance and be competitive in any sport. Speed and agility are two closely related skills needed for most sports. There are some good athletes, such as a junior varsity football running back, who have tremendous speed but lack the agility to make multiple cuts to get away from defenders and gain yards. Likewise, there are athletes, such as a nationally ranked high school tennis player, who have great agility to change directions laterally but not enough speed to chase down a volley to the outside corner of the court. Athletes who work equally as hard in these two areas will greatly increase their chances of dominating their competitors.

# Speed Drills

Speed is the ability to gain maximal acceleration in the shortest amount of time possible. Speed endurance, as in running a 400 meter race, involves maintaining an optimal speed over an extended period of time. Much of our speed is genetic, as some people are just born with a greater number of fast twitch muscle fibers than others. Fast twitch fibers are the muscle fibers that have a limited supply of blood and oxygen, and they are specifically designed for short burst activities requiring power and strength (such as sprinting). This is in contrast to slow twitch muscle fibers, which are heavily saturated with blood and oxygen. Slow twitch fibers are good for endurance activities where there is a higher demand of oxygen. Although there is a certain genetic makeup for each person, an athlete can train to become faster by training those fast twitch muscles that are available. This requires anaerobic exercise, which is different from aerobic exercise. Anaerobic activities last no longer than 60 sec, and many would argue that the time is much less than that. It emphasizes activation of fast twitch muscle fibers, as opposed to the slow twitch fibers that are activated with aerobic activity where the goal is endurance. The goal of anaerobic training is to reduce the build-up of lactic acid that is acquired with short bouts of fast twitch activation. This is what causes muscle cramping with sprints.

Speed training requires more than just running sprints. However, sprints are essential in creating those fast twitch gains. The length of the sprint depends on the demand of the sport. Football players generally do not have to run more than 40 yards at a time, but they play on a 100 yard field. Therefore, alternating between shorter sprints up to 40 yards and longer sprints up to 140 yards will be optimal. In track and field, sprinters train for speed endurance by doing sprints that are longer than their event. This helps them to hold that top speed throughout the duration of the race. For example, a 100 meter sprinter may frequently run 150-200 meter sprints to train his or her fast twitch muscles anaerobically to hold that speed without cramping from lactic acid buildup. For athletes competing in sports that require very short bursts of speed, such as in volleyball or tennis, shorter sprints would be fine. In sports that do not require running, such as figure skating and boxing, speed training can be beneficial to build anaerobic tolerance with sport specific activities (punching, twisting and spinning on the ice).

Starts, quick foot strikes from a high knee position, high knees, and butt kicks are common speed drills that can be performed inside or outside. If equipment is available or if there is funding for equipment, there are several good options. Speed parachutes and dual-attachment bungee cords are great for working on speed with resistance. Weight-adjustable speed sleds are also very good for training speed with resistance, and also improving power.

When performing resistance exercises to improve speed, athletes should be trained with a balance between strength and power. General strength is needed, as well as muscle hypertrophy, to increase the size of the muscles and fast twitch muscle fibers. However, to improve turnover, or the ability to drive the feet off the ground and duplicate that running pattern more quickly, power exercises are needed. Some specific power exercises that can be incorporated into the resistance program include, but are not limited to, hang cleans, dead lifts, and power squat jumps. Keep in mind that sprinting is a full body activity, so strengthening the upper body is also important. Examples of upper extremity exercises include bench press, back rows, shoulder circuits, and biceps/triceps curls and extensions with dumbbells.

# Agility Training

Agility is the ability to perform change of direction movements, and to change the speed at which these movements are performed. Agility is what allows a soccer player to sprint down the sideline with the ball, then stop "on a dime" and cut toward the middle of the field to aim and kick the ball into the goal. It's what allows a basketball player to perform a crossover move followed by a spin to shake her defender and, with a burst of speed, drive to the basket to score. Agility requires a certain amount of strength to perform these movements efficiently without placing too much force and stress on the joints, which can lead to injury. Additionally, neural adaptations within the brain and within the muscles have to be trained to improve the athlete's ability to make decisions about change of speed and direction movements, and then to take action on these decisions and carry out those movements.

Speed ladder drills are a great way to improve agility. There are a number of activities that can be performed using the speed ladder, from forward/backward to lateral movements, and changing directions. Hopping and jumping using the speed ladder is also effective, and should be performed in both double leg and single leg fashion. Cutting activities with cones, such as the "T drill", are also effective agility drills. The greater the number of directions performed with these drills, the greater the gains in agility. Therefore, it is not enough just to perform these activities in a linear motion, such as forward or lateral. Athletes should also be trained in diagonal planes and backward, which allows for greater adaptations to the neural pathways in the brain and trains the muscles to react to stresses in multiple directions. If an athlete shows a significant weakness on one side, or is returning from injury, it is essential to perform these activities unilaterally to reduce compensatory strategies that may develop.

Regarding resistance training, power exercises are the best way to help train the muscles to respond to changes in direction and speed. Again, cleans, squats, and dead lifts are great power exercises. Bench press, clean and jerks, snatches, and push-ups with a hand clap are also excellent explosive exercises. By adding weights, the muscles are trained to not only improve strength, but also the ability of the muscles to increase the speed of changing from an elongated position to a contracted position. This is the underlying neurologic adaption needed to improve agility.

As stated earlier, strength and agility complement each other. Gains in one area can improve the performance in the other. There is also much overlap in the type of resistance training needed to increase gains in speed and agility. There is a saying that "speed kills", meaning that speed trumps strength and size. However, speed with agility trumps everything! Being able to control one's speed, decelerate quickly, cut and change direction, then accelerate quickly is the best weapon any athlete can have. Lastly, training must include emphasis on technique and form in order to prevent injuries since these types of activities place a high stress demand on the body.

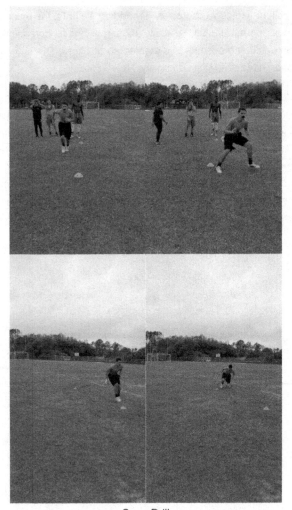

Cone Drill

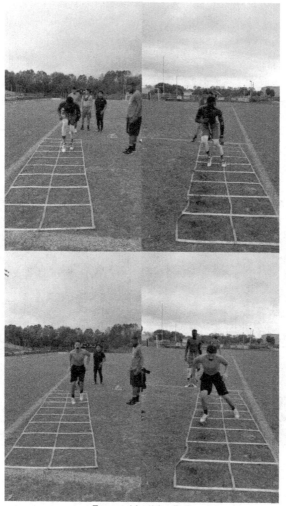

Forward Ladder Drill

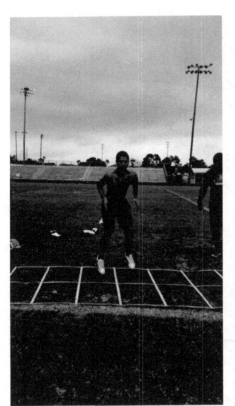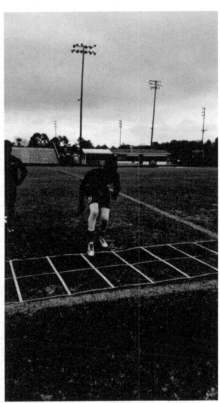

Lateral Ladder Drill

# 8

# BALANCE AND CORE

Balance and core strengthening are often grossly overlooked when formulating conditioning programs for youth athletes. The two also go hand in hand just as speed and agility drills complement each other. Improving core strength will help to improve functional balance, just as training on balance will help to improve core strength.

# Balance

What is it that allows us to keep from falling when we stumble? How is a wide receiver able to make a great catch on the sideline and run to the end zone without stepping out of bounds? What keeps a gymnast so still and eloquent in her movements while twirling and flipping on a 6 inch wide beam? The answer is balance. Balance is the way the body is able to find itself in space and maintain a centered, upright position. There are three components to balance—vision, cerebellar righting, and somatosensory. The first two are completely related to the eyes and brain. The last, somatosensory balance, is directly related to neurologic signals that are sent to the body's extremities from the brain. The largest component of the somatosensory system is proprioception, or how the body uses these nerve signals to find its position in space at any given time. These sensors are found throughout the body's extremities, mostly in the feet but also in the hands and throughout the joints of the lower extremities.

As with speed, everyone is born with a specific genetic makeup of balance. However, balance can also be improved with proper training. This is especially important for athletes who are returning from injury. Single leg balance is a great way to work on balance, and to determine if someone has an imbalance unilaterally. Changing the surface on which the athlete is standing will change the level of difficulty. For example, standing on a foam pad will be more challenging that on a flat surface, and standing on a Bosu ball will be more challenging than foam. Things to watch when training balance are differences between the left and right sides, hyperextension of the knees, increased flexion (bending) at the hips, arms reaching outward as if to catch oneself, and increased swaying back and forth at the trunk. These are all compensatory strategies to make up for a lack of balance starting at the feet and ankles, or it may be a sign of core weakness (or both).

Another key component to improving balance is strengthening. As the muscles surrounding the joints of the body are strengthened, this increases the stability of the joints, thus improving the proprioceptive responses needed for balance. The concept of single leg balance can be applied when performing resistance exercises. Single leg squats, single leg straight leg dead lifts with a dumbbell, and standing straight leg kicks with a resistance band are great examples of single leg balance activities. For double leg activities, one can incorporate balance by changing the surface. Performing squats while standing on a Bosu ball is a good example. I actually prefer to do single leg squats on the Bosu (black side up) when I work on balance, and it is a great way to activate the gluteals and hamstrings more. The athlete can also perform walking lunges with a trunk twist, or single leg calf raises are other ways to improve balance.

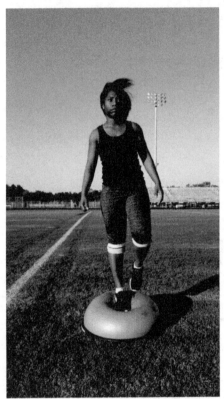
Single Leg Balance on
Bosu

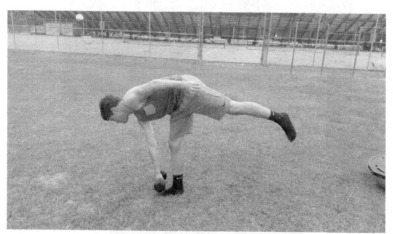

Single Leg Dead Lift With
Dumbbell

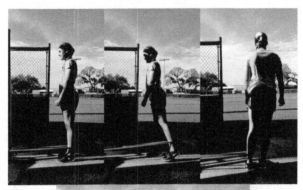

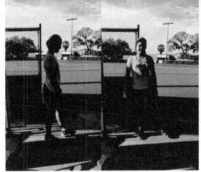

4-Way Kicks With
Resistance Band

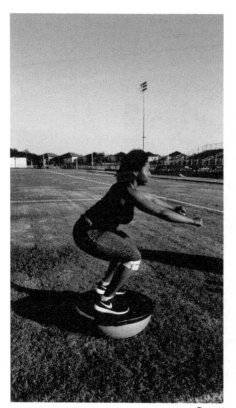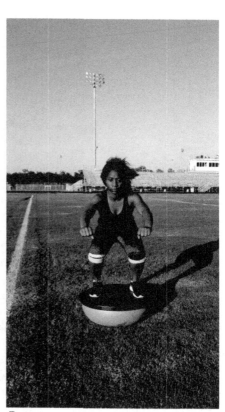

Squats on Bosu

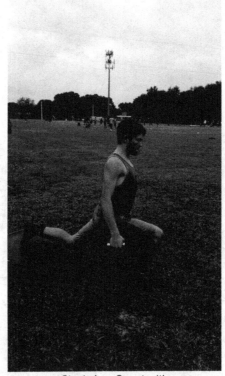

Single Leg Squat with
Back Leg on Bosu

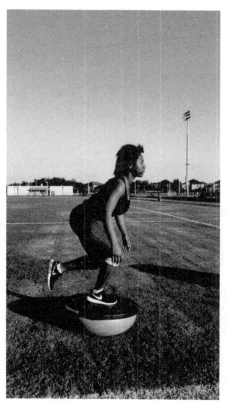

Single leg Squat on Bosu

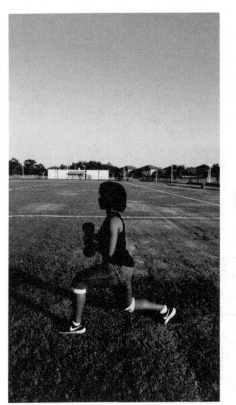 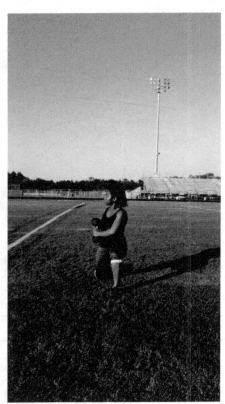

Walking Lunge With Trunk
Twist

# Core Strengthening

Another key component to stabilization in the body, one that can also affect an athlete's balance, is the core. Most people only associate the abdominal muscles with the term "core". However, it also includes the pelvic floor muscles, and the muscles of the thoracic and lumbar spine regions. The back stabilizers are important in keeping the body upright in sitting and standing, and the abdominals counterbalance and keep the body from falling backward. Any imbalance in abdominal or back stabilizer strength can create abnormal movement patterns with functional activities such as running, squatting, throwing, and jumping.

There are many ways to strengthen the core other than regular sit ups and curl ups. In fact, for an athlete who has a history of back pain, these exercises are typically not recommended. One of my favorite exercises to strengthen the core is planks. A more beneficial way to do planks, one that is less stressful to the back, is to do side planks, with the athlete on a bent elbow and the entire body raised off of the mat (except the feet). Most athletes, especially younger athletes, have weak cores. Moreover, they have weakness in the lateral core and oblique abdominal and lumbar musculature. Side planks address this area of weakness. Better exercises to work the abdominals without creating increased stress on the back are those that involve the lower extremities moving or being pulled toward the trunk. Examples include V-ups, bicycles, and mountain climbers. If using an exercise ball, place the athlete face down toward the mat, with elbows extended, and legs on the ball. Then, draw the knees into the chest while keeping the hips down as low as possible (plank with double knee to chest). This exercise is great to engage the lower abdominals and activate the hip flexors in the groin region.

When addressing the posterior side of the core (the thoracic and lumbar muscles), there are different strategies. Bridges are an essential exercise to gaining posterior core strength. Not only do bridges engage the lower lumbar muscles, they also facilitate activation of the gluteals and hamstrings. Adding an exercise ball under the legs helps to activate the abdominals, and a progression to bringing the knees to the chest using the ball will help to engage the hamstrings more. Quadruped exercises are also good for the posterior core, with the athlete starting on hands and knees. Supermans, an exercise involving alternating arm and leg lifts while in quadruped, activates the muscles close to the spine to improve stability with upright (standing or sitting) activity.

Core activation can be implemented into resistance training with many of the common strengthening exercises. For instance, performing biceps curls in a sit-up position is a great way to work the arms while engaging the abdominals. Performing push-ups with the hands on a Bosu ball is another great upper extremity exercise. Doing a bench press using dumbbells while the athlete has the top of his or her back on an exercise ball vs doing traditional bench press on a flat bench, will engage the core. Relating to lower extremity exercises, resistance bands with side steps, lunges, and squats can help activate the lower pelvic floor muscles and abdominals. The band should be placed either around the ankles or just above the knees. Coaches and trainers can also help athletes learn to engage their core with all lifting exercises by giving verbal cues to keep the belly tucked in tight before performing the repetition.

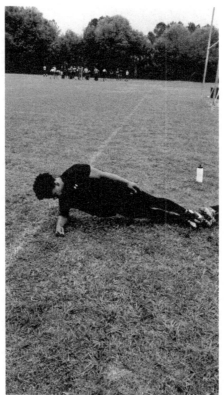

Side Plank

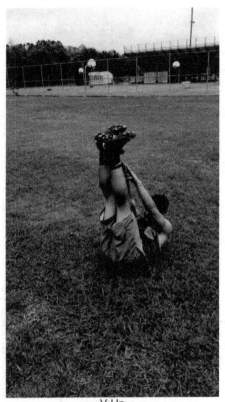

V-Up

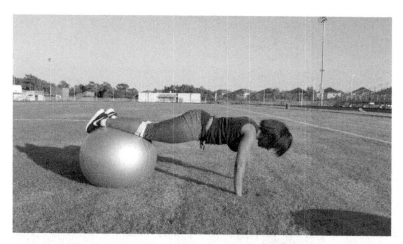

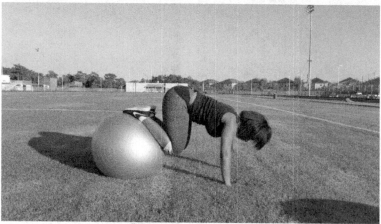

Plank With Double Knee
to Chest

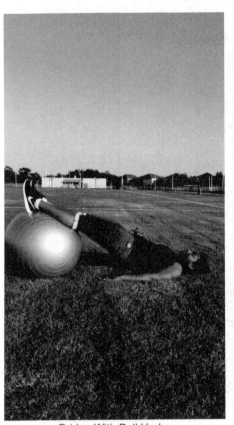

Bridge With Ball Under
Legs

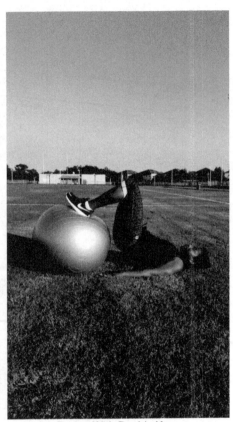

Bridge With Double Knee
to Chest

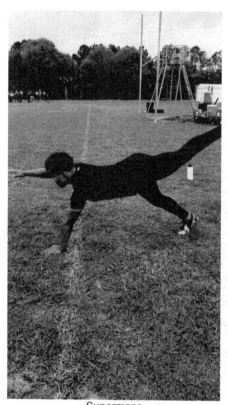

Supermans

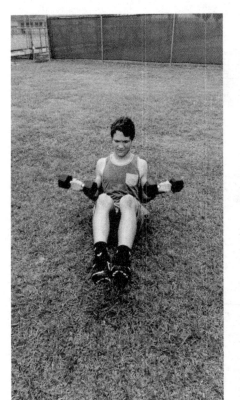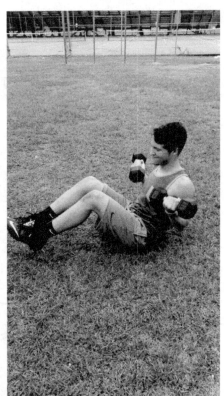

Biceps Curls in Sit-up
Position

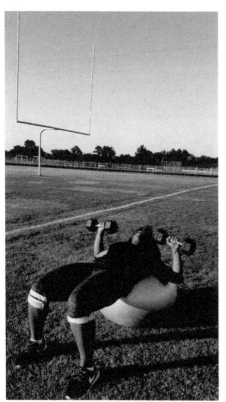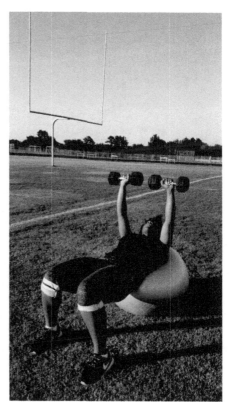

Dumbbell Press on Ball

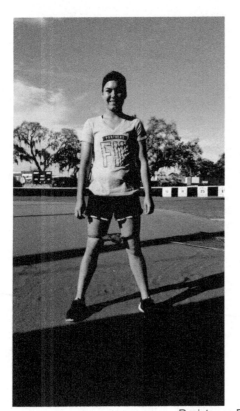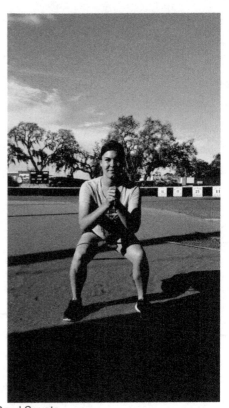

Resistance Band Squats

# 9

# PLYOMETRICS AND HIIT EXERCISES

The last two components to a well-balanced training program are plyometric (or plyos) and HIIT exercises. These two components both involve high intensity and high stress loads on the body. They should be used as a complement to the other components of training, and should not be performed every day.

# Plyometrics

The term plyometric ("plyos") means any exercise that involves activating the highest level of force in a given muscle in the shortest amount of time. This places a very high demand on the muscles, similar to resistance exercises to gain power. There is something called amortization time, the time in which a muscle changes from a stretched position to a contracted position. The goal of plyometric exercise is to decrease this time as much as possible, which helps to improve power, agility (change in direction), and speed.

Medicine ball activities are a great way to work on plyometric conditioning. Medicine ball push pass with partners, medicine ball slams on the floor, and power squats with a medicine ball toss are just a few examples. Box jumps, step off squat jumps, bounding, continuous double leg jumps, and standing broad jumps are examples of lower extremity plyos. In addition to medicine ball activities, weighted ball toss with a rebounder (trampoline), and push-ups with a hand clap are examples of plyos for the upper extremities. Speed ropes can also be used for upper extremity plyos, but they usually involve a total body movement with initiation of power and force coming through the lower extremities. Plyometric exercises for the upper extremities are not as common as plyos for the lower extremities.

Due to the explosiveness of the exercises and the load stress on the muscles and joints, certain considerations must be taken into account when performing plyometric drills. Children who have not yet started, or who have just started puberty, should only be doing plyometric exercises sparingly. Athletes who have been injured should be progressed to plyos only once their pain has been managed, and they have adequate strength and ROM to perform the movements safely. When conducting plyometric exercises, qualified coaches and trainers need to closely monitor body mechanics and posture with each athlete to ensure there is no risk of injury. For example, if the knees turn inward towards each other while performing a step down squat jump, this is an unsafe posture. Girls will be more likely to exhibit this posture than boys. Symmetry is also important when assessing form, making sure the athlete is landing on both feet with the weight distributed evenly between the right and left.  Similarly, when performing upper extremity plyos such as a medicine ball toss, it is important to make sure the athlete is using a chest pass with both arms pushing equally as he or she steps forward to follow through the motion.

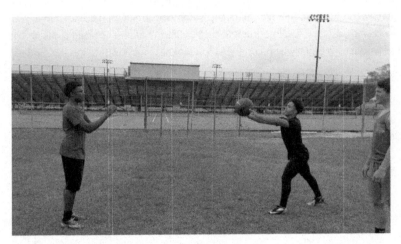

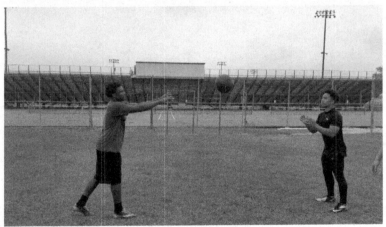

Medicine Ball Toss

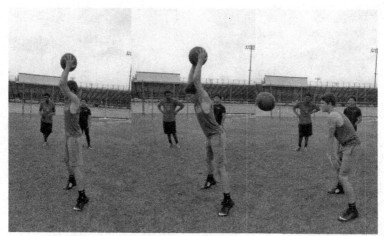

Medicine Ball Slam

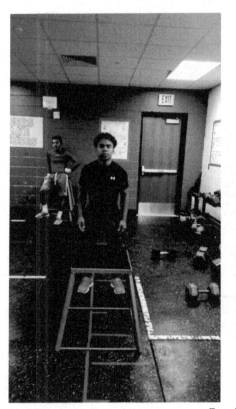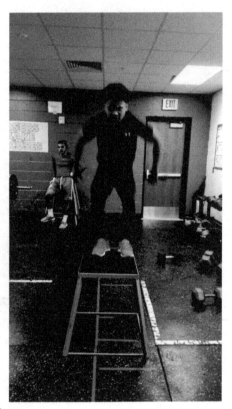

Box Jump

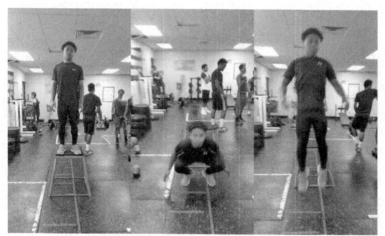

Step Down Squat Jump

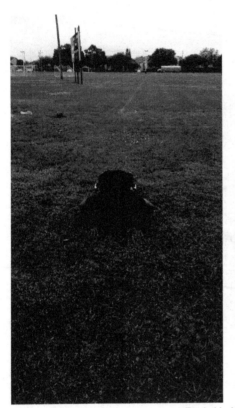 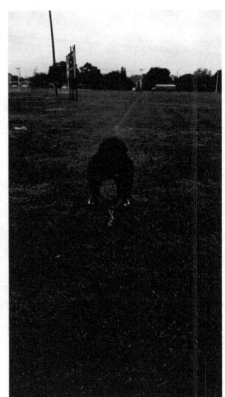

Push-Up With a Clap

# HIIT Exercises

The term HIIT has been used more frequently in the past couple years. It stands for High Intensity Interval Training. This can include performing many of those plyometric exercises discussed earlier, but for a longer duration. The purpose of HIIT training is to strengthen the muscles in a plyometric fashion while incorporating an aerobic component to the activity. Each activity is typically performed from 30-60 seconds in a round robin or circuit format, usually consisting of 4 to 5 exercises. Each round or circuit is performed 2 to 3 times. While some muscle groups can be targeted with specific exercises, HIIT training is typically a way to get a "full body" workout in one session. A great example of this is the Burpee exercise, which has become very popular on sports teams all across the country.

An example of a HIIT circuit would be high knees in place, squat jumps, mountain climbers, plank jacks, and alternating lunge jumps. Each exercise is performed for 30 seconds, continuing on to the next exercise without stopping to rest. Once the circuit is complete, a small rest may be given, about 60 seconds, and the circuit is repeated. In the example circuit, the exercises chosen are predominantly lower extremity exercises, with high knees, squat jumps, and lunge jumps. However, a "break" is given in the middle of the circuit while the athlete performs mountain climbers and plank jacks, which will activate the core and work the arms.

HIIT training is great to do in groups, and can be used as an alternative or complement to resistance training. Coaches in colder climates like to use HIIT training on cold rainy/snowy days when they are not able to practice outside. It is more difficult to keep track of form and posture when working with groups of athletes performing different circuits at the same time. However, detailed explanation and demonstration of each exercise before starting a circuit can help minimize injuries from poor mechanics and form. Because HIIT drills carry more of a cardio element than plyos, they are safer to perform with younger athletes. However, caution should always be observed when training kids pre-pubescent or at the start of puberty.

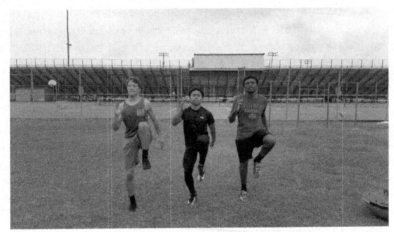

High Knees in Place

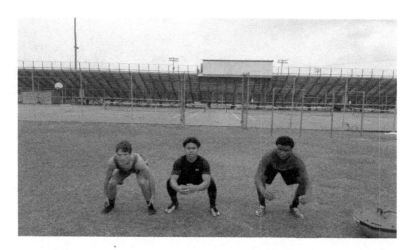

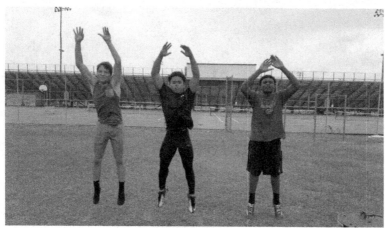

Squat Jumps

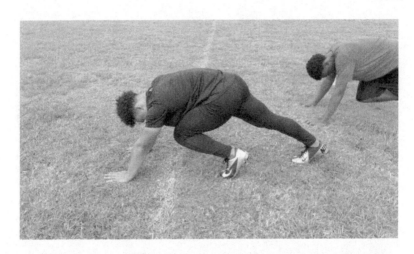

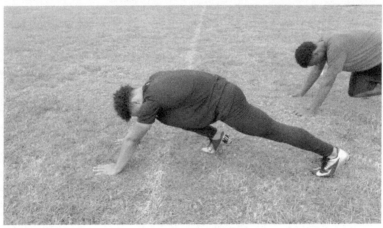

Mountain Climbers

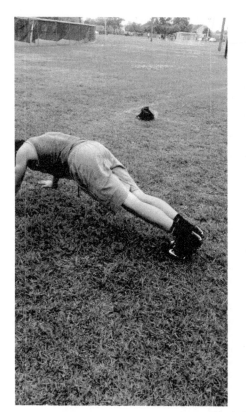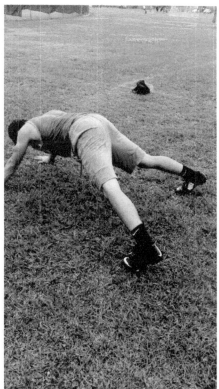

Plank Jacks

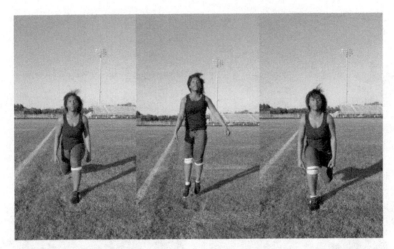

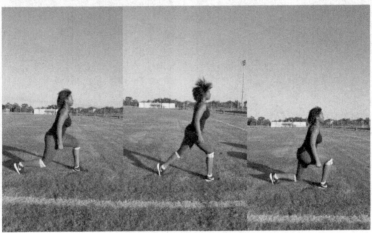

Alternating Lunge Jumps

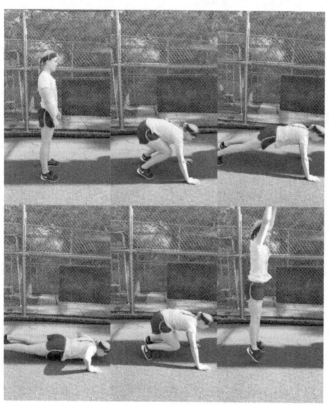

Burpees

# 10
# PERIODIZATION

The question that coaches frequently ask is directly related to periodization. Periodization is a term used to describe the sequence and methods for organizing a training schedule for a specific sport. This training schedule will include all of the areas that have been discussed previously, in addition to any sport specific requirements. Timing of each component along with the changes in intensity of training are vital to the performance of the athlete, and are essential in reducing the likelihood of injury. There are also differences in training schedules before the season starts, during the season, and after the season.

# Pre-Season Preparation

Before the sport season begins (the "off-season"), a heavy emphasis should be placed on aerobic and resistance training. This is the time to work on the cardiovascular improvements that occur within the body with prolonged aerobic training. The biggest strength gains can also be made when the athletes do not have to worry about a competition every week. Cardio exercise times may be longer, up to 45-60min, and resistance repetitions may be higher to achieve strength and hypertrophy gains. Cross-training is a good way to build cardiovascular benefits. For example, if an athlete participates in track and field, having him or her participate in swimming and biking for their aerobic exercise in addition to running will help to build endurance and the necessary adaptations more quickly. HIIT exercises are also another great way to incorporate cardio exercise into the workouts. This is not to say that plyometric agility exercises will not be performed at all during this period, but the emphasis is on restoring and improving strength and cardiovascular endurance. This portion of the preparation phase can last from 12-16 weeks.

The next portion of the preparation phase usually starts about 4-6 weeks from the beginning of the season. Sport specific drills will start to ramp up, as well as speed, agility, and plyometric activities. Resistance training will now emphasize power exercises vs strength/hypertrophy. Medicine balls, speed ladders, running sleds, parachutes, and bungee cords are excellent tools for speed, agility and plyometric training. During the first part of the off-season, resistance training may be incorporated up to 6 times per week. However, in the second half of the preparation season resistance training should be tapered down to 3-4 times per week. Aerobic training will also be tapered down to 3-4 times per week vs 6. Scrimmages, trial performances, and mock meets will also begin during this period. The intent of these practice runs is to tailor training progression and correct any deficiencies in sport-specific skills.

# In-Season Training

This part of the training cycle is the period in which competitions begin. Athletes can finally put their hard work and training to good use and battle opponents with the hopes of victory! In many sports, performance may not be as great in the beginning of the season as it is at the end during higher level and more elite competitions. This is because there is usually a "peaking" cycle for the sport that, if cycled properly, should have the athletes at their best toward the end of the season when championship rounds approach. This is best seen in the sport of track and field, where athletes expect to see their times decrease with each meet, and their personal best times occur at the end of the season at championship meets.

Ideally, a typical week of training during competition season will include one day of high intensity training, two days at moderate to high intensity, one light to moderate, and one low intensity day. It is best to have the low intensity day the day before competition. There is debate as to whether or not to exercise the day after competition. In my opinion, I believe that this should be a full day without exercise, especially for sports that are very physically demanding, such as football. However, if any exercise is done it should be low intensity.

Typically, if a sport's "in-season" is longer than 3 months, there needs to be a "rest" period about every 4-5 weeks in which the intensity level of training is taken down to low or low to moderate. This allows the athletes to recharge and prevent fatigue and injuries. In sports with seasons lasting less than 3 months, there may only be one of these low intensity cycles. All of the components to training may still be implemented during the season, with a heavy emphasis on sport specific drills and simulation. For sports that have more than one season (spring and fall, or winter and spring, etc), there will be multiple cycles of varying intensity training.

# Overtraining

Many coaches get wrapped up into maximizing the intensity during each training session without any periods of rest or low intensity. Without this break, fatigue and injury are inevitable. The human body can only maintain peak performance for so long, and if it is pushed beyond this threshold the results are deleterious, not beneficial. Young athletes are even more susceptible to fatigue and breakdown in the body that occurs with overtraining. Younger athletes may still be going through puberty, and may still be growing. Taking on increased stress loads to the joints and muscles at constant high intensity can permanently damage the growth process. This is why adequate rest, sleep, and periodic transitions to low intensity training are necessary. If the athlete has to take time to go to the doctor or physical therapy due to an injury, she is not able to perform in her sport. Having to rehab frequent or chronic injuries also makes it very difficult to increase the level of intensity of training when needed.

# Post-Season

Once the competition season reaches its close, a period of "off-season" begins. Depending on the sport, this can last anywhere from 4 weeks to 6 months. The initial 1-2 weeks should be dedicated to rehab of injuries, rest and recovery from a trying season. Unless the athlete is recovering from an injury, this post-season period must include, at a minimum, aerobic and resistance training at low to moderate intensity, with the goal of preventing deconditioning. Occasional drills and sport specific activities can also be included. If an off-season lasts up to 6 months, the preparation period before starting the in-season needs to begin at least 3 months prior to the start of the season. In sports with shorter off-seasons, training intensity may be reduced to low to moderate through the majority of the off season, with a short rest period the week immediately following completion of competition to allow for healing and recovery.

# 11

# CONCLUSION

Improving performance in youth athletes is not just about physical performance. There are a number of components involved, beginning with mindset. With proper mental toughness, an athlete is capable of achieving much more than coaches, family, friends, and naysayers can imagine. A collaborative effort is needed to ensure the athlete is well aware of things that can be done to decrease the risk of injury, and ensure that a long number of years of sport are ahead if desired. It is important to also understand that training to be competitive in a sport goes far beyond warming up, doing a few push-ups, and going out to play. There are specific strategies that can be included into a training program to maximize the athlete's cardiovascular endurance, strength, power, speed, and agility. Knowing how and when to implement these training components can make or break the performance and success of the athlete.

# Thank You

First and foremost, I would like to thank God, for without You none of this would be possible. I would like to thank my parents, Richard and Randy Stokes, for teaching me invaluable lessons and for making me the woman I am today. My brother, Jason Stokes, a phenomenal athlete and coach, and a great mentor to young athletes for many years. To my cousin/brother Brian Bennett, whose gifts are immeasurable. The world is ready for you to unlock your full potential! To all of my former coaches in all of the sports in which I've competed. I am grateful that all of you dedicated yourselves to helping me achieve more success than I could have imagined, success that transcended to all of facets of my life. I also want to give special thanks to a dear friend, Dr. Siobhan France, who has taught me to do more than just be strong enough to survive. You have inspired me to be great and to create success that provides significance to many peoples' lives. Lastly, to all of my family and friends who have supported me through all of my endeavors, thank you!

For the photos, I would like to thank all of the amazing athletes who helped me with those awesome shots! Thank you to the members of the Gaither High School football team, including Adam, Jordan, Deante, Kyle, David (D-Rod), Elijah, and Coach Rex. I would also like to thank Talicia (LeLe) and Madison for the great action shots!

# About the Author

*My name is Dr. Amy E. Stokes and I am a Doctor of Physical Therapy originally from Ft. Washington, MD. I graduated from the United States Naval Academy in 2003 with a Bachelor of Science degree in Chemistry. After serving two years as an Ensign in the United States Navy, I decided to make a change from serving my country as a whole, to serving my community at large. I began Physical Therapy school and graduated from the University of Miami in 2008 with a Doctor of Physical Therapy degree (DPT). While in PT school, I also passed the national exam and earned my Certified Strength and Conditioning Specialist (CSCS) certification. I have maintained an active status since 2007. As a Physical Therapist, I have worked in both permanent and contract positions throughout the DC metro area, in a variety of settings, but primarily in an outpatient setting with an orthopedic population. I am currently practicing in the Tampa, FL area. My experience as a CSCS extends from managing a youth baseball camp in Miami, to working with patients one on one and in group boot camp settings both individually and in association with Elite Fitness Pros in Washington, DC.*

*My love for sports and fitness began at age 5 when I started on my first soccer team. The ball came up to my knees but I was the most determined and fearless one out on the field! At age 10, I found my true love in track. I was a middle distance runner, competing in everything from the 400m to 400m hurdles, and up to the 800m and 1500m. My track career lasted through my 4 years at the Naval Academy, and I've received many awards from Patriot League Champion, to holding a spot in my school record book that stands to this day. In 2009, I decided to become a "weekend warrior" and began playing in a competitive flag football league in the Washington, DC area. Most recently in February 2015, I began training to compete in bodybuilding as a Figure model, and I was crowned the 2015 Maryland State Champ.*

*Throughout my many competitions and successes on the athletic field, I have had to deal with several injuries and surgeries, including an ACL repair in 2009 and a medial meniscus tear in 2011. Those were just reminders to me that I had to maintain the maximum level of fitness possible for me to enjoy the things I love to do. My time in the military has definitely helped keep me on a structured regiment that allows me to perform at an optimal level of fitness. My constantly improving knowledge of injury prevention, rehab, and the latest techniques in strength training have only enhanced my health and wellness.*

*I love having the opportunity to work with clients/patients from different levels of fitness and medical status, from post-op knee scopes to elite level runners who want to improve core strength. The age group I enjoy working with the most are the student athletes from ages 10-18, because I was once a student athlete and will always remember the amazing coaches and trainers I had at that time. I enjoy being able to teach students about injury prevention and giving them the latest training techniques to improve their performance and see them develop into great athletes. My hope is that this book can and will be used as a tool for athletes, coaches, and parents while on their quest to achieve greatness!*

*To contact me, please email me at stokesamye@yahoo.com, or on Facebook (Amy Stokes).*

*Coming soon... www.dramyestokes.com which will be my official business website and blog page.*

Made in United States
North Haven, CT
13 June 2022

20219138R00055